CW00517734

Anti-Inflammatory Eating Made Easy

Delicious and Healthy Cookbook

Linda J. Hebert

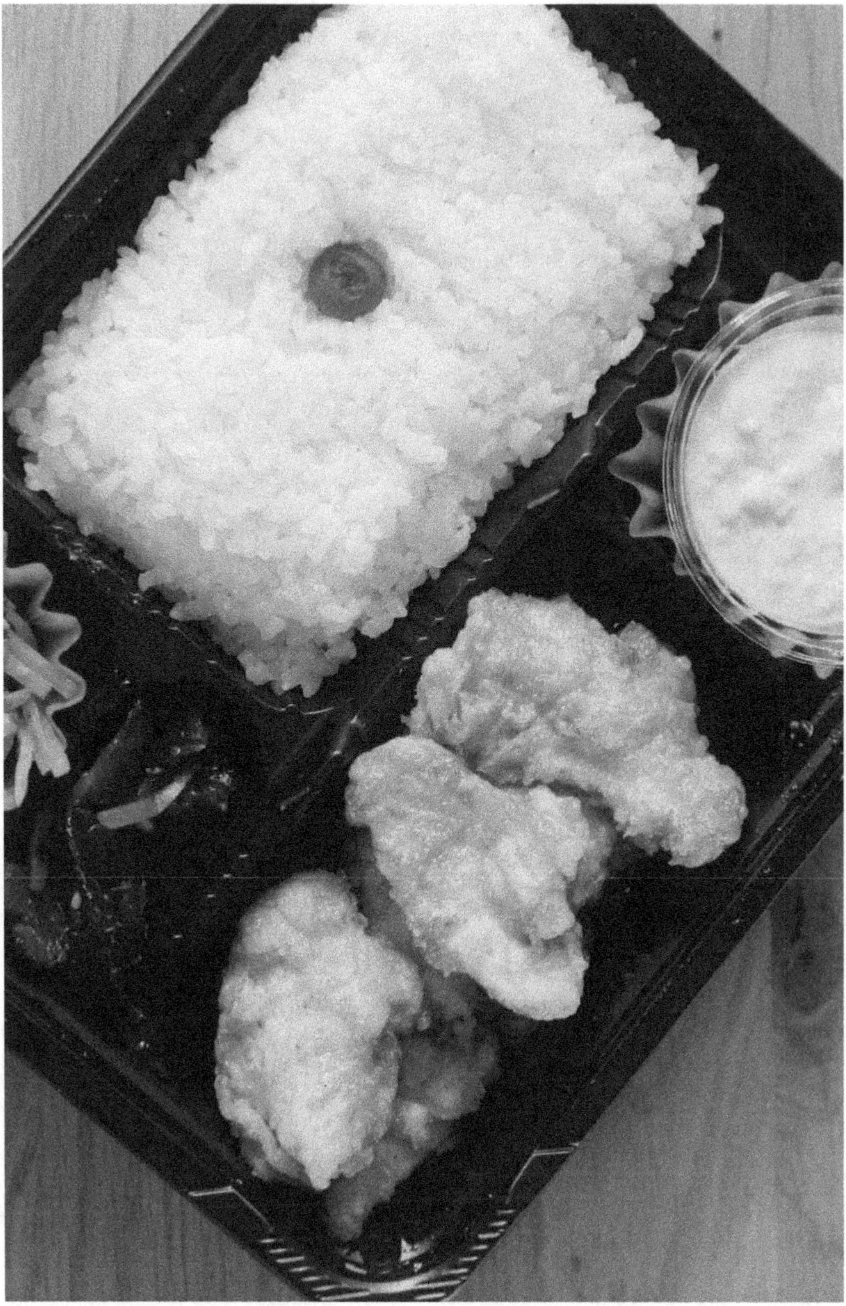

Table of Contents

Introduction

An anti-inflammatory diet favors fruits and vegetables, foods containing omega-3 fatty acids, whole grains, lean protein, healthful fats, and spices. It discourages or limits the consumption of processed foods, red meats, and alcohol. The anti-inflammatory diet is not a specific regimen but rather a style of eating.

This book will help you with tasty recipes!

Spinach & Berries Smoothie
Pineapple & Carrot Smoothie

A great refreshing smoothie using the tasty flavor of pineapple and

carrot. This recipe makes a real delightful

smoothie. Yield: 2 servings

Preparation Time: 10 minutes

Ingredients:1 cup frozen pineapple

1 large ripe banana, peeled and sliced

½ tablespoon fresh ginger, peeled and chopped

¼ teaspoon ground turmeric

1 cup unsweetened almond milk

½ cup fresh carrot juice

1 tablespoon freshly squeezed lemon juiceDirections:

1. In a high-speed blender, add all ingredients and pulse till smooth.

2. Transfer into 2 glasses and serve immediately.

Nutritional Information per Serving:

Calories: 144, Fat: 2.3g, Carbohydrates: 32g, Fiber: 5g, Protein: 2.4g

Nutty Berries & Spinach Smoothie

A super smoothie. This smoothie is loaded with all the healthy kale

and sweet distinct taste of fresh berries in addition to their juices.

Yield: 3 servings

Preparation Time: 10 min

Ingredients:¾ cup frozen blackberries

¾ cup frozen blueberries

1 frozen banana, peeled and sliced

1 cup fresh baby spinach

¼ cup raw walnuts

1 teaspoon bee pollen

1½ cups unsweetened almond milkDirections:

1. In an increased speed blender, add all ingredients

and pulse till smooth.

2. Transfer into 2 glasses and serve immediately.

Nutritional Information per Serving:

Calories: 115, Fat: 0.5g, Carbohydrates: 18g, Fiber: 4.3g, Protein: 2.1g

Cherry & Kale Smoothie

Treat one's body with one of delicious and juice smoothie. Cherries,

kale and banana create a nice combo with spices.

Yield: 1 serving

Preparation Time: 10 minutes

Ingredients:2 ripe bananas, peeled and sliced

1 cup fresh cherries, pitted 1 cup fresh kale,

trimmed

1 teaspoon fresh ginger, peeled and chopped

1 tablespoon chia seeds, soaked for 15 minutes

½ teaspoon ground turmeric

¼ teaspoon ground cinnamon

1 cup coconut waterDirections:

1. In a top speed blender, add all ingredients and pulse

till smooth.

2. Transfer in a glass and serve immediately.

Nutritional Information per Serving:

Calories: 103, Fat: 0.6g, Carbohydrates: 13g, Fiber: 5.2g,

Protein: 2.2g

Veggies & Turmeric Smoothie

One from the best and smoothies that has multiple healing qualities.

Avocado adds a superbly creamy touch with this smoothie.

Yield: 2 servings

Preparation Time: 10 minutes

Ingredients:1 small avocado, peeled, pitted and chopped

½ of green bell pepper, seeded and chopped

1-inch fresh turmeric piece, peeled and grated

1 cup fresh baby spinach, chopped

1 cup fresh arugula, chopped

1-inch fresh ginger piece, peeled and chopped

¾ cups fresh parsley

Pinch of cayenne

Pinch of salt

1 cup fresh coconut waterDirections:

1. In a top speed blender, add all ingredients and pulse till smooth.

2. Transfer into 2 glasses and serve immediately.

Nutritional Information per Serving:

Calories: 115, Fat: 0.4g, Carbohydrates: 19g, Fiber: 9.1g, Protein: 12.2g

Banana & Ginger Smoothie

A great addition in their email list of healthy smoothies. This smoothie

is full of the flavor of naturally healthy ginger and banana.

Yield: 1 serving

Preparation Time: 10 min

Ingredients:1-inch fresh ginger piece, peeled and

chopped 1 frozen banana, peeled and sliced

½ teaspoon ground cinnamon

1 cup coconut milkDirections:

1. In a higher speed blender, add all ingredients and pulse

till smooth.

2. Transfer in to a glass and serve immediately.

Nutritional Information per Serving:

Calories: 110, Fat: 0.6g, Carbohydrates: 22g, Fiber: 5.7g, Protein: 10.2g

Pineapple, Kale & Ginger Smoothie

One of your nutrient-dense smoothies. This smoothie is a fantastic

way to bring along in a lot of nutrients as well as in your

daily diet.

Yield: 1 serving

Preparation Time: 10 min

Ingredients:1 cup frozen pineapple, chopped 1 tablespoon fresh ginger, peeled and chopped

1 cup fresh kale, trimmed and chopped

½ cup fresh mixed berries

¼-½ teaspoon ground turmeric, to taste

2 teaspoons ground flax seeds

1 cup unsweetened coconut milk

½ cup ice, crushedDirections:

1. In a higher speed blender, add all ingredients and pulse till smooth.

2. Transfer into 1 glass and serve immediately.

Nutritional Information per Serving:

Calories: 121, Fat: 0.1g, Carbohydrates: 25g, Fiber: 10.1g, Protein: 20.2g

Pineapple & Green Tea Smoothie

A simple tasty recipe of smoothie while using flavors of pineapple

and teas. This recipe prepares a really energizing and delicious

smoothie.

Yield: 1 serving

Preparation Time: 10 min

Ingredients:1 cup pineapple, chopped

1 small little bit of ginger, peeled and chopped

½ teaspoon ground turmeric

1 teaspoon natural immune support

1 teaspoon chia seeds

1 cup cold teas

½ cup Ice, crushedDirections:

1. In an increased speed blender, add all ingredients and pulse till smooth.

2. Transfer in a glass and serve immediately.

Nutritional Information per Serving:

Calories: 121, Fat: 0g, Carbohydrates: 11g, Fiber: 9.1g, Protein: 1.2g

Fruit & Veggie Smoothie

A freshest and quickest way to obtain veggies and fruit in your daily

diet in the same time. This blend makes a really yummy smoothie.

Yield: 2 servings

Preparation Time: fifteen minutes

Ingredients:¾ cups pineapple, chopped

½ cup cucumber, peeled and chopped

½ of pear, peeled, cored and chopped

1 small avocado, peeled, pitted and chopped

½ tablespoon fresh dill

1 cup fresh spinach, chopped

1 celery stalk, chopped

¼ teaspoon ground turmeric

1-piece fresh ginger, peeled

1 tablespoon fresh lime juice

2 cups waterDirections:

1. In a top speed blender, add all ingredients and pulse till

smooth.

2. Transfer into 2 glasses and serve immediately.

Nutritional Information per Serving:

Calories: 130, Fat: 0.1g, Carbohydrates: 25g, Fiber: 10.1g, Protein: 20.0g

Spiced Peach Smoothie

A really delicious and healthy smoothie recipe using a kick of warm

spices. This natural mix of peaches and spices is really a refreshing,

cool summertime smoothie.

Yield: 2 servings

Preparation Time: 10 minutes

Ingredients:½ of frozen banana, peeled and

chopped 1 cup frozen peaches, pitted and chopped

½ teaspoon ground ginger

½ teaspoon chia seeds

1 teaspoon ground turmeric

1 teaspoon ground cinnamon

1 teaspoon raw honey

10-ounce unsweetened almond milkDirections:

1. In a higher speed blender, add all ingredients and pulse till smooth.

2. Transfer right into a glass and serve immediately.

Nutritional Information per Serving:

Calories: 99, Fat: 0g, Carbohydrates: 16g, Fiber: 6.4g, Protein: 15.2g

Tangy Mango & Spinach Smoothie

One of smoothie with refreshing lemony touch. This smoothie is

actually light, healthy and refreshingly

delicious. Yield: 2 servings

Preparation Time: 10 minutes

Ingredients:2 cups frozen mango, peeled, pitted and chopped

3 cups fresh spinach, chopped

1 teaspoon ground turmeric

16-ounce fresh coconut water

1 tablespoon fresh lemon juice

1 tablespoon lime juiceDirections:

1. In a high-speed blender, add all ingredients and pulse

till smooth.

2. Transfer into 2 glasses and serve immediately.

Nutritional Information per Serving:

Calories: 111, Fat: 0g, Carbohydrates: 25g, Fiber: 9.3g, Protein: 16.4g

Pineapple, Avocado & Spinach Smoothie

A smoothie while using healthy nutrients of pineapple, spinach and

avocado. Fresh cilantro adds a really nice taste in this smoothie.

Yield: 2 servings

Preparation Time: 10 minutes

Ingredients:¼ of pineapple, peeled and

chopped 3 cups spinach, chopped

¼ of avocado, peeled, pitted and chopped

¼ cup fresh cilantro, chopped

½-inch fresh ginger piece, peeled and

chopped 1 tablespoon chia seeds

1 tablespoon ground turmeric

Fresh cracked black pepper, to tasteDirections:

1. In a high-speed blender, add all ingredients and pulse till smooth.

2. Transfer right into a glass and serve

immediately. Nutritional Information per Serving:

Calories: 122, Fat: 0g, Carbohydrates: 20g, Fiber: 12.3g,
Protein: 21.2g

Kale & Avocado Smoothie

A smoothie with power blending ingredients. You can get best tasting

healthy nutrients in this simple smoothie.

Yield: 2 servings

Preparation Time: 10 min

Ingredients:3 stalks fresh kale, trimmed and chopped

1-2 celery stalks, chopped

½ of avocado, peeled, pitted and chopped

½-1 ginger herb, chopped

½-1 turmeric root, chopped

2 cups coconut milkDirections:

1. In a higher speed blender, add all ingredients and pulse

till smooth.

2. Transfer into 2 glasses and serve immediately.

Nutritional Information per Serving:

Calories: 137, Fat: 0.4g, Carbohydrates: 20g, Fiber: 12.3g, Protein: 29.2g

Strawberry & Beet Smoothie

A healthy combo of strawberries, beet, fresh ginger and fresh

turmeric. Fresh orange juice adds a delish citrus taste.

Yield: 2 servings

Preparation Time: 10 minutes

Ingredients:2 cups frozen strawberries, pitted and chopped

2/3 cup roasted and frozen beet, chopped 1 teaspoon

fresh ginger, peeled and grated

1 teaspoon fresh turmeric, peeled and grated

½ cup fresh orange

juice 1 cup almond milk

Directions:

1. In a top speed blender, add all ingredients and pulse

till smooth.

2. Transfer into 2 glasses and serve immediately.

Nutritional Information per Serving:

Calories: 133, Fat: 0.1g, Carbohydrates: 24g, Fiber: 12.5g, Protein: 24.2g

Pineapple & Orange Smoothie

A smoothie with all the combo of sweet pineapple and citrus. This

incredibly simple smoothie is wonderful for

kids. Yield: 1 serving

Preparation Time: 10 minutes

Ingredients:1 fresh orange, peeled and chopped

1½ cups fresh pineapple, chopped

1 small thumb of ginger, peeled and chopped/grated

1 frozen banana, peeled and sliced

1 teaspoon ground turmeric

1 tablespoon chia seeds

1 cup unsweetened almond milkDirections:

1. In a higher speed blender, add all ingredients and pulse till smooth.

2. Transfer in a glass and serve immediately.

Nutritional Information per Serving:

Calories: 123, Fat: 0g, Carbohydrates: 14g, Fiber: 11.2g, Protein: 19.2g

Anti-Inflammatory Eating Made Easy

Pineapple & Coconut Smoothie

One from the tasty smoothie with tropical dream. The combo of

pineapple and coconut gives this smoothie such a light and refreshing

flavor.

Yield: 1 serving

Preparation Time: 10 minutes

Ingredients:1 cup fresh pineapple,

diced 1 tablespoon coconut, shredded

½ lime, peeled and seeded

1 tablespoon chia seeds

1 teaspoon ground turmeric

Pinch of freshly ground black pepper

½ cup coconut waterDirections:

1. In a high-speed blender, add all ingredients and pulse till smooth.

2. Transfer in a glass and serve immediately.

Nutritional Information per Serving:

Calories: 130, Fat: 0.2g, Carbohydrates: 26g, Fiber: 7.2g, Protein: 17.4g

Pineapple & watermelon Smoothie

One with the refreshing smoothie with sweet and citrus flavoring.

This refreshing smoothie is satisfying and delicious.

Yield: 2 servings

Preparation Time: 10 min

Ingredients:1 cup frozen pineapple, chopped

1 fresh orange, peeled and sliced (white pith and seeds removed)

2 cups frozen watermelon, peeled, pitted and chopped

1 teaspoon fresh ginger, peeled and chopped

½ teaspoon ground turmeric

½ cup coconut milk

1 teaspoon organic honey

1½ cups coconut waterDirections:

1. In a higher speed blender, add all ingredients and pulse till smooth.

2. Transfer into 2 glasses and serve immediately.

Nutritional Information per Serving:

Calories: 122, Fat: 0g, Carbohydrates: 23g, Fiber: 5g, Protein: 16.1g

Pineapple & Mango Smoothie

Such a wonderfully delicious smoothie. Surely, you'll have the real

taste of tropics in this smoothie.

Yield: 1 serving

Preparation Time: 10 min

Ingredients:2¼ cups mixed mango and pineapple, peeled and

chopped

1 tablespoon chia seeds

1 teaspoon ground turmeric

½ teaspoon ground ginger

½ teaspoon ground cinnamon

Pinch of vanilla powder

1 cup coconut milk

1 teaspoon coconut oilDirections:

1. In a higher speed blender, add all ingredients and pulse

till smooth.

2. Transfer into a glass and serve immediately.

Nutritional Information per Serving:

Calories: 127, Fat: 0g, Carbohydrates: 28g, Fiber: 2.1g, Protein: 22.2g

Cherry & Blueberry Smoothie

A sweet smoothie with a creamy texture. It will probably be perfect

for a delicious breakfast or snack treat.

Yield: 1 serving

Preparation Time: 10 min

Ingredients:2 cups escarole

½ cup frozen blueberries

½ cup frozen cherries

¼ teaspoon ground cinnamon

¼ teaspoon ground turmeric

1 scoop of chocolate Protein powder

1 cup filtered water

5 ice cubes, crushedDirections:

1. In an increased speed blender, add all ingredients

and pulse till smooth.

2. Transfer in a glass and serve immediately.

Nutritional Information per Serving:

Calories: 126, Fat: 0g, Carbohydrates: 26g, Fiber: 12g,

Protein: 15g

Berries, Watermelon & Avocado Smoothie

A delicious smoothie using a creamy texture without the use of any

dairy. Avocado provides a creamy base to the smoothie.

Yield: 1 serving

Preparation Time: 10 minutes

Ingredients:1½ cups mixed frozen berries

1 cup watermelon, peeled, seeded and chopped

¼ avocado, peeled, pitted and chopped

1-inch fresh ginger piece, peeled and chopped

2 teaspoons chia seeds

¾ cup fresh coconut waterDirections:

1. In a high-speed blender, add all ingredients and pulse till

smooth.

2. Transfer into a glass and serve immediately.

Nutritional Information per Serving:

Calories: 146, Fat: 0.1g, Carbohydrates: 27g, Fiber: 12.4g, Protein: 32.4g

Pear, Peach & Papaya Smoothie

A fabulous smoothie with the flavors of three fruit blend. This

smoothie is incredibly healthy too.

Yield: 3 servings

Preparation Time: 10 min

Ingredients:½ cup pear, peeled, cored and chopped

¾ cup peaches, pitted and chopped

¾ cup papaya, peeled and chopped

1 teaspoon fresh ginger, peeled and chopped

2 fresh mint leaves

½ cup coconut water

1 cup ice, crushedDirections:

1. In an increased speed blender, add all ingredients

and pulse till smooth.

2. Transfer into 3 glasses and serve immediately.

Nutritional Information per Serving:

Calories: 158, Fat: 0g, Carbohydrates 14.5g, Fiber: 13g, Protein: 27g

Apple, Strawberry & Beet Smoothie

A blend of bright red ingredients. Make this smoothie for the family

and receive huge applause.

Yield: 4 servings

Preparation Time: 10 min

Ingredients:2 cups frozen strawberries, hulled and sliced

1 beet, peeled and chopped

1 cup apple, peeled, cored and sliced

3 Medjool dates, pitted and chopped

¼ cup extra virgin coconut oil

½ cup unsweetened almond milkDirections:

1. In an increased speed blender, add all ingredients

and pulse till smooth.

2. Transfer into a glass and serve immediately.

Nutritional Information per Serving:

Calories: 173.4, Fat: 0.6g, Carbohydrates: 22.3g, Fiber: 6.9g, Protein:

2.2g

Cherry & Beet Smoothie

A smoothie that will certainly give you a blast of energy. Cherries,

berries, beets and avocado complement the other person very nicely.

Yield: 1 serving

Preparation Time: 10 minutes

Ingredients:¾ cup frozen pineapple, chopped

1 cup frozen berries

¼ cup frozen red beets, peeled and chopped

¼ small avocado, peeled, pitted and chopped

1 tablespoon chia seeds

1 teaspoon fresh ginger, peeled and chopped

½ teaspoon fresh turmeric, grated

2 teaspoons raw honey

1 cup unsweetened almond milkDirections:

1. In a high-speed blender, add all ingredients and pulse till smooth.

2. Transfer in a glass and serve immediately.

Nutritional Information per Serving:

Calories: 195, Fat: 0.8g, Carbohydrates: 24g, Fiber: 10.4g, Protein: 32g

Spiced Banana Smoothie

A healthy, sweet and thick smoothie with healthy spices. This banana

smoothie is a full meal alone.

Yield: 1 serving

Preparation Time: 10 min

Ingredients:2 bananas, peeled and sliced

2 teaspoons ground ginger

½ teaspoon ground turmeric

½ teaspoon organic vanilla

flavor 1 tablespoon honey

1 cup coconut milk

6-8 ice cubes, crushedDirections:

1. In a high-speed blender, add all ingredients and pulse

till smooth.

2. Transfer right into a glass and serve

immediately. Nutritional Information per Serving:

Calories: 199, Fat: 0g, Carbohydrates: 25g, Fiber: 12.8g, Protein: 19g

Pineapple & Almond Smoothie

Incredibly delicious smoothie with frothy texture. Surely this

smoothie would be kids friendly.

Yield: 3 servings

Preparation Time: 10 minutes

Ingredients:1 cup fresh pineapple, peeled and chopped

¼ cup blanched almonds ½

cup fresh pineapple juice ½

teaspoon pure maple syrup

½ cup fresh pineapple juice

¼ cup rice milk

½ cup ice cubes, crushedDirections:

1. In a top speed blender, add all ingredients and pulse

till smooth.

2. Transfer in to a glass and serve immediately.

Nutritional Information per Serving:

Calories: 96.7, Fat: 5.2g, Carbohydrates: 11.6g, Fiber: 1.3g, Protein: 2.5g

Papaya & Pineapple Smoothie

A smoothie while using tastes of fresh pineapple and papaya. This

refreshing and nutritious smoothie can be a hit for a morning treat.

Yield: 1 serving

Preparation Time: 10 minutes

Ingredients:1½ cups pineapple, peeled and chopped

½ of papaya, peeled and chopped

2 dates, pitted

1½ cups coconut waterDirections:

1. In a higher speed blender, add all ingredients and pulse

till smooth.

2. Transfer in a glass and serve immediately.

Nutritional Information per Serving:

Calories: 237, Fat: 0g, Carbohydrates: 60g, Fiber: 4g, Protein: 3g

Watermelon, Berries & Avocado Smoothie

A delicious smoothie with all the refreshing taste of summer. This

smoothie is good for hot summer days.

Yield: 1 serving

Preparation Time: 10 minutes

Ingredients:1½ cups mixed frozen berries

1 cup watermelon, peeled, seeded and chopped

¼ of avocado, peeled, pitted and chopped

1-inch fresh ginger piece, peeled and chopped

2 teaspoons chia seeds

¾ cup fresh coconut waterDirections:

1. In a top speed blender, add all ingredients and pulse

till smooth.

2. Transfer right into a glass and serve

immediately. Nutritional Information per Serving:

Calories: 177, Fat: 1g, Carbohydrates: 20g, Fiber: 13g, Protein: 26.5g

Cherry & Pineapple Smoothie

This smoothie can be a good way to pack the nutrition inside your

kid's diet. Surely your kids would love to love this particular

smoothie

Yield: 1 serving

Preparation Time: 10 min

Ingredients:¼ of pineapple, peeled and

chopped 12 fresh cherries, pitted

¼ of beetroot, peeled and chopped

1 tablespoon chia seeds

1 cup coconut water

½ cup ice, crushedDirections:

1. In a high-speed blender, add all ingredients and pulse till

smooth.

2. Transfer in to a glass and serve immediately.

Nutritional Information per Serving:

Calories: 150, Fat: 4.5g, Carbohydrates: 21g, Fiber: 10g, Protein: 6g

Nutty Banana & Ginger Smoothie

A powerhouse smoothie while using combo of banana, nuts and

healthy seeds with fresh turmeric and cinnamon. This smoothie will

likely be ideal for kids.

Yield: 4 servings

Preparation Time: 10 min

Ingredients:1 frozen banana, peeled and

sliced ¼-inch fresh turmeric root, grates

½-inch fresh ginger root, peeled and chopped

1 cup pecans, chopped

1 cup walnuts, chopped

1 tablespoon flax seeds

1 tablespoon chia seeds

1 tablespoon fresh maca powder

½ teaspoon ground cinnamon

1½ cups unsweetened almond milkDirections:

1. In a high-speed blender, add all ingredients and pulse till

smooth.

2. Transfer into 4 glasses and serve immediately.

Nutritional Information per Serving:

Calories: 193, Fat: 1g, Carbohydrates: 25g, Fiber: 9g, Protein: 11.2g

Pineapple, Mango & Coconut Smoothie

A wonderful smoothie that combines pineapple, mango, coconut and

Goji berries greatly. This smoothie is delicious and healthy at the same

time.

Yield: 2 servings

Preparation Time: 10 min

Ingredients:1 cup pineapple, chopped

½ cup mango, peeled, pitted and chopped

Flesh and water of your coconut

1 tablespoon Goji berries

½ teaspoon fresh turmeric, chopped

1 teaspoon chia seeds

1 cup brewed teasDirections:

1. In a higher speed blender, add all ingredients and pulse

till smooth.

2. Transfer into 2 glasses and serve immediately.

Nutritional Information per Serving:

Calories: 203, Fat: 1.2g, Carbohydrates: 24g, Fiber: 5.3g, Protein: 32g

Tangy Avocado & Ginger Smoothie

A super nutritious and delicious smoothie. This delicious smoothie

also looks beautiful using its vibrant blue color.

Yield: 1 serving

Preparation Time: 10 min

Ingredients:½ cup frozen berries

2 tablespoons unsweetened coconut, shredded

1/3 cup low- Fat cottage cheese

1 packet stevia

8-ounce coconut water

½ cup ice, crushedDirections:

1. In a top speed blender, add all ingredients and pulse

till smooth.

2. Transfer in a glass and serve immediately.

Nutritional Information per Serving:

Calories: 175, Fat: 2.4g, Carbohydrates: 19g, Fiber: 13g, Protein: 19g

Tangy Ginger & Radish Smoothie

A wonderful approach to enjoy healthy ingredients in your smoothie.

This smoothie comes with ginger punch and fresh citrus flavor.

Yield: 2 servings

Preparation Time: 10 minutes

Ingredients:1 orange, peeled, seeded and

sliced 1 radish, trimmed and chopped

1 tablespoon fresh ginger, peeled and chopped

5-10 fresh mint leaves

1 tablespoon ground chia seeds

1 teaspoon organic honey

1 cup spring water

½ cup fresh orange juice

1 tablespoon freshly squeezed lemon juice

Ice, as required

Directions:

1. In a higher speed blender, add all ingredients and pulse

till smooth.

2. Transfer into 2 glasses and serve immediately.

Nutritional Information per Serving:

Calories: 212 Fat: 0g, Carbohydrates: 25g, Fiber: 13g, Protein: 177g

Sweet Potato & Orange Smoothie

A simple delicious smoothie which is packed with healthy nutrients of

sweet potato, orange and ginger. orange juice adds a refreshing touch

within this smoothie.

Yield: 2 servings

Preparation Time: 10 min

Ingredients:1 medium banana, peeled and

sliced 1 cup sweet potato puree

1 teaspoon fresh ginger, chopped

½ tablespoon flax seeds meal 1

tablespoon almond butter ¼

teaspoon ground turmeric ¼

teaspoon ground cinnamon ¾

cup unswee10ed almond milk

¼ cup fresh orange juice

Ice, as requiredDirections:

1. In an increased speed blender, add all ingredients and

pulse till smooth.

2. Transfer into 2 glasses and serve immediately.

Nutritional Information per Serving:

Calories: 189, Fat: 0.1g, Carbohydrates: 27g, Fiber: 3g, Protein: 12g

Strawberry & Kale Smoothie

One of the great breakfast smoothies having a little citrus touch.

Strawberries and kale combines greatly with this smoothie.

Yield: 1 serving

Preparation Time: 10 min

Ingredients:½ fresh strawberries, hulled and

sliced 1 cup fresh kale, trimmed and chopped 1

celery stalk, chopped

½ of lime, peeled

1 cup coconut waterDirections:

1. In a higher speed blender, add all ingredients and pulse till smooth.

2. Transfer in a glass and serve immediately.

Nutritional Information per Serving:

Calories: 234, Fat: 0g, Carbohydrates: 20g, Fiber: 9g, Protein: 17g

Blueberry & Cucumber Smoothie

A quick and healthy blueberry smoothie. Banana adds a natural

sweetness to this healthy smoothie recipe.

Yield: 1 serving

Preparation Time: 10 min

Ingredients:½ cup cucumber, peeled and chopped

½ of small banana, peeled and

sliced 1 cup frozen blueberries

1 tablespoon chia seeds

1 cup waterDirections:

1. In a top speed blender, add all ingredients and pulse till smooth.

2. Transfer in to a glass and serve immediately.

Nutritional Information per Serving:

Calories: 213, Fat: 0g, Carbohydrates: 27g, Fiber: 6g, Protein: 1.2g

Carrot Soup

A great strategy to consume fresh carrots in what you eat. This bright,

citrusy and nourishing soup is packed with great

texture. Yield: 8 servings

Preparation Time: 15 minutes Cooking Time: 1 hour

40 minutes Ingredients:2-pounds carrots, peeled and

cut into slices 7 tablespoons extra-virgin essential olive

oil, divided 2 large fennel bulbs, sliced

Salt, to taste

¼ cup pumpkin seeds

1 medium yellow onion, chopped

6 garlic cloves, minced

1 tablespoon fresh ginger, grated

1 tablespoon ground turmeric

½ teaspoon red pepper cayenne

2 tablespoons fresh lime juice

1½ cups coconut milk

4-6 cups water

¼ cup scallion (green part), mincedDirections:

1. Preheat the oven to 375 degrees F.

2. In a baking sheet, place the carrot and drizzle with 2 tablespoons of oil.

3. Roast approximately one hour.

4. Remove the carrots from oven and make aside.

5. Now, raise the temperature of oven to 400 degrees F.

6. In a skillet, heat 3 tablespoons of oil on medium heat.

7. Add fennel bulbs and pinch of salt and sauté for about 4-5 minutes.

8. Transfer the fennel bulb onto a baking sheet and roast approximately 20-a half-hour.

9. Meanwhile, heat a nonstick skillet on medium heat. Keep aside.

10. Add pumpkin seeds and stir fry for around 3-4 minutes or till toasted. Keep aside.

11. Meanwhile in a very soup pan, heat remaining oil on medium heat.

12. Add onion and sauté for around 12 minutes.

13. Add garlic and sauté for approximately 1 minute.

14. In a blender, add onion mixture, carrots, ginger, spices, lime juice and coconut milk and pulse till well combined.

15. Add required amount of water and pulse till smooth.

16. Return the soup in the pan on medium heat.

17. Bring to some boil and cook approximately 3-5 minutes.

18. Serve hot with all the topping of fennel and pumpkin seeds.

Nutritional Information per Serving:

Calories: 230, Fat: 16g, Carbohydrates: 20g, Fiber: 6g, Protein: 5g

Carrot & Ginger Soup

A flavorful bomb for a healthy and delicious meal. This soup is often a

great strategy to use fresh carrots and ginger in your

meal. Yield: 4 servings

Preparation Time: 15 minutesCooking Time: 30 minutes

Ingredients:1 tablespoon coconut oil 1 medium brown

onion chopped

2 minced garlic cloves

1 long red chili, chopped

1 (1/3-inch) fresh turmeric piece, peeled and sliced

1 (¾-inch) fresh galangal piece, peeled and sliced

1 (¾-inch) fresh ginger piece, peeled and sliced

4 cups carrots, peeled and chopped

2 lemongrass stalks

2 cups water

2 cups vegetable broth

Coconut cream, as requiredDirections:

1. In a substantial soup pan, heat oil on medium heat.

2. Add onion and sauté for about 5 minutes.

3. Add garlic, red chili, turmeric and sauté for approximately 5 minutes.

4. Add carrots, lemongrass stalks, water and broth and produce to some boil.

5. Reduce the warmth to low and simmer for about 15-20 minutes.

6. Remove from heat and aside to chill slightly.

7. Discard the lemongrass stalks.

8. In a blender, add soup in batches and pulse till smooth.

9. Serve immediately with the topping of coconut cream. Nutritional Information per Serving:

Calories: 299, Fat: 7g, Carbohydrates: 25g, Fiber: 12g, Protein: 18g

Curried Carrot & Sweet Potato Soup

A filling soup using the flavors of vegetables. This pureed soup is

really a wonderful strategy to take pleasure in the flavors of sweet

potato and carrot.

Yield: 5 servings

Preparation Time: 15 minutes

Cooking Time: 37 minutes

Ingredients:2 teaspoons olive oil

½ cup shallots, chopped

1½ cups carrots, peeled and sliced into ¼-inch size

3 cups sweet potato, peeled and cubed into ½-inch size

1 tablespoon fresh ginger, grated

2 teaspoons curry powder

3 cups Fat-free chicken

broth Salt, to tasteDirections:

1. In a sizable soup pan, heat oil on medium heat.

2. Add shallots and sauté for approximately 3 minutes.

3. Add carrot, sweet potato, ginger and curry powder and sauté for around 3-4 minutes.

4. Add broth and bring to a boil.

5. Reduce heat to low.

6. Cover and simmer approximately 25-thirty minutes.

7. Stir in salt and black pepper and remove from heat.

8. Keep aside to cool down the slightly.

9. In a blender, add soup in batches and pulse till smooth.

10. Serve immediately.

Nutritional Information per Serving:

Calories: 131, Fat: 2.1g, Carbohydrates: 23.1g, Fiber: 3.9g, Protein: 5.7g

Creamy Broccoli Soup

A healthy and delicious soup recipe with creamy texture. Avocado

supplies the creamy touch to the delicious soup.

Yield: 3-4 servings

Preparation Time: 15 minutes

Cooking Time: 35 minutes

Ingredients:1 tablespoon virgin coconut

oil 1 celery stalk, chopped

½ cup white onion, chopped

Salt, to taste

1 teaspoon ground turmeric

2 minced garlic cloves

1 large head broccoli, cut into florets

¼ teaspoon fresh ginger, grated

1 bay leaf

1/8 teaspoon cayenne pepper

Freshly ground black pepper, to

taste 5 cups vegetable broth

1 small avocado, peeled, pitted and chopped

1 tablespoon fresh lemon juiceDirections:

1. In a substantial soup pan, heat oil on medium heat.

2. Add celery, onion and several salt and sauté for around 3-4 minutes.

3. Add turmeric and garlic and sauté for approximately 1 minute.

4. Add desired mount of salt and remaining ingredients except avocado and lemon juice and provide with a boil

5. Reduce heat to medium-low.

6. Cover and simmer for about 25-thirty minutes.

7. Remove from heat and keep aside to cool down the slightly.

8. In a blender, add soup and avocado in batches and pulse till smooth.

9. Serve immediately with the drizzling of freshly squeezed lemon juice.

Nutritional Information per Serving:

Calories: 275, Fat: 3g, Carbohydrates: 20g, Fiber: 13g,

Protein: 28g

CPSIA information can be obtained
at www.ICGtesting.com
Printed in the USA
BVHW090631270421
605864BV00004B/768

9 781802 325270